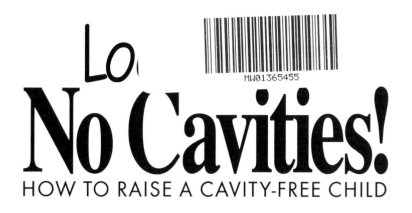
Look No Cavities!
HOW TO RAISE A CAVITY-FREE CHILD

Gregory F. George, D.D.S.

First Edition

A Publication Of:

Look Mom...No Cavities!

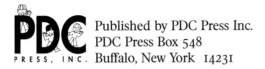

Published by PDC Press Inc.
PDC Press Box 548
Buffalo, New York 14231

Copyright © 1998 by Gregory F. George, D.D.S.
All Rights Reserved
Edited by Jordana Halpern Geist
Design by John D. Valerio, White & Company Inc.

First edition 1998

ISBN #: 0-9662475-0-7

Without limiting the rights under copyright alone, no part of this publication may be reproduced, stored in or introduced into a retrieval system, or transmitted in any form or by any means (electronic, mechanized, photocopying, recording or otherwise) without the prior written permission of both the copyright owner and the above publisher of this book.

Printed in the U.S.A.

For information on PDC Press Books and other products, including sales inquires and special prices for bulk quantities, write to the address above, or contact PDC Press, Inc. at 1-888-292-1991.

For general information and news updates visit our website at www.lookmom.com

This publication is directed towards young children and parents concerned about dental health. Hopefully, the information contained herein will be useful and helpful to them. However, it should not be viewed as dental advice and readers should understand that the author and publisher are not rendering professional dental services to them. Readers should consult their personal dentist about their individual dental health care. The author, publisher and all other persons associated with this publication disclaim any liability arising out of, or relating to, any reliance upon information contained in this publication.

Acknowledgements

A SPECIAL THANKS TO EVERYONE WHO HELPED ME WITH THIS BOOK:

My father, who always encouraged me to reach for the stars and to help other people.

My mother, who taught me the Golden Rule and that we can do and be anything we really want if we want it enough.

My stepmother, who taught me about unconditional love and selflessness.

My wife and children, who were patient enough to allow me to write this book and whose love on a daily basis fills my life.

The wonderful group of people I work with at Pediatric Dental Care, who make every day at work fun.

Andy White and John Valerio, for their work on layouts, illustrations, printing, ideas and honesty.

Deborah Smith, for her help with jacket design and book style.

Judie Takacs and Maria Walczak, for their support and encouragement to bring this project to fruition.

Jordana Halpern Geist, for her enthusiasm, guidance, knowledge and great editing skills.

Michael Morrone, for his editorial input.

Finally I wish to thank the thousands of patients, parents and friends in my dental practice, who have taught me so much.

In memory of
Frank T. George

Contents

INTRODUCTION - THE GOAL: 100% CAVITY-FREE	8
1. THE BENEFITS OF CAVITY PREVENTION	12
2. THE BATTLE BETWEEN TEETH AND BACTERIA	16
3. THE DANGERS OF TOOTH DECAY	22
4. FIGHTING BACK - THE WAR AGAINST BACTERIA	28
5. FOOD - THE GOOD, THE BAD AND THE UGLY	36
6. GIVING NATURE A HAND	44
7. CONCLUSION - MAKING OUR GOAL A REALITY	52
8. CHECK LISTS FOR CAVITY PREVENTION	56

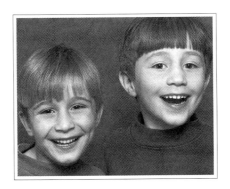

INTRODUCTION

The Goal:
100% Cavity-Free

Raising cavity-free children can be an attainable, realistic goal for all parents. All that is required is a little extra care and use of an easy-to-follow program that requires less than ten minutes a day.

DEAR PARENTS:

As the father of young children, I share your dream of raising healthy children.

Like so many other busy parents, my wife and I seem to be constantly sifting through mountains of advice to determine the best way to achieve this goal. Just as we think we have something figured out, a completely new report appears the following day. It's hard to know what's right.

Fortunately, there is an important area of our children's health where we can gain control, and that is our children's teeth. I am proud to say that our children have never had a cavity and I am confident they never will. As a pediatric dentist with a large and successful practice dedicated to minimizing cavities in children, I would like to share with you a simple, effective program to help you raise cavity-free children.

Do you remember as a child, feeling a tingling or painful shooting sensation when chewing on bubble gum or chocolate? Maybe you remember the buzz of the drill grinding into your jawbone as the dentist cleaned out cavities.

If you follow the practical advice in this book, your child will never need to experience those painful or frightening sensations. All that is required is a little extra care and use of the knowledge that I want to share with you.

Follow these basic guidelines and your child will never have to hide a painful tooth under their tongue while eating something cold or sweet. Your toddler will not lose front teeth at three years of age or have to live with large black fillings. Your child will not need to chew on one side of his mouth to avoid pain or be teased about bad breath caused by dental decay. And your child may not have to deal with braces, made necessary because a tooth was removed early due to decay.

THE CAVITY-FREE PLAN

In the following pages, I'll show you how to teach your child skills and habits that they can carry through their lives and pass on to their own children.

It's a plan that shows you how to keep your children's teeth cavity-free with good dental hygiene and preventative treatments to strengthen tooth enamel. And, it's an easy-to-follow program that requires less than ten minutes a day.

Because your child's diet is a major factor in their dental health, I will also discuss the role that different foods play in cavity formation. This is an area over which you have tremendous control. Offering your child the right

INTRODUCTION

foods and avoiding bad foods will also prevent decay of their teeth.

Finally, we'll discuss how establishing a relationship with a caring dentist can enhance your efforts in raising a cavity-free child. If your child's dentist has not yet seen this book, please feel free to highlight any points you may want to share.

The ideas and techniques in this book will work for most children. Unfortunately, there will always be some children whose teeth grow in with structural defects or with cavities already formed. Some children inherit genetic traits that make them more susceptible to decay. Although these children may require additional services, the information in this book will help reduce their chances for developing cavities.

You've already taken a positive step by picking up this book. Now I ask you for about an hour of your time. It's a small investment to make in exchange for the healthy smile you'll see on your child's face for many years to come.

Sincerely,

Gregory F. George, D.D.S.

1 0 0 %   C A V I T Y - F R E E

CHAPTER ONE

The Benefits Of Cavity Prevention

From a very early age, children become conscious of their appearance. Healthy teeth play an important role in every child's self-image and self-confidence levels. A healthy smile immediately attracts positive attention from neighbors, teachers, peers and other family members.

It used to be accepted that losing teeth was a normal part of the aging process. Denture creams and cleansers were a common sight in household medicine cabinets, as was the image of gleaming teeth sitting in a glass by the bedside.

But technology and attitudes have changed. Now we know that most of us can keep our teeth for a lifetime. And keeping our teeth offers many positive benefits.

We can maintain healthier, more diverse diets. Because our teeth naturally support facial muscles, we can maintain a younger appearance. We will save time and money avoiding denture fittings and cleanings. Let's face it – it's much more convenient to use the teeth already in our

THE BENEFITS OF CAVITY PREVENTION

mouth, rather than put them in and take them out each day.

FILLINGS – A SECOND BEST SOLUTION

It's true that the current choices for repairs are many and growing. But as far as we've come with technology, it is still much better to avoid getting a cavity in the first place.

We're still waiting for the perfect filling material to be invented. Some fillings wear faster than real teeth. Others expand, shrink or are sensitive to hot or cold temperatures. Some will fall out as the sealer or glue dissolves away over time. Still others crack after excessive, repeated chewing.

We also want to avoid cavities, because once the decayed part of the tooth is removed, the remaining tooth is structurally weaker. A restored tooth will have a seam where the filling and tooth join. And this region will be more prone to future breakdown than a natural tooth.

Even though most fillings today are totally painless, the reality is, that your child will never confuse a cavity-filling session with a trip to the amusement park. Fillings today may be quick and easy, but they often involve a local anesthetic such as Novocaine™, or a relaxing gas such as nitrous oxide, also known as laughing gas.

And let's not forget the inconvenience for children who miss school or extracurricular activities, and for the parents who often miss work while their children's teeth are being restored.

APPEARANCES COUNT

From a very early age, children become conscious of their appearance. Healthy teeth play an important role in every child's self-image and self-confidence levels. A healthy smile immediately attracts positive attention from

CHAPTER ONE

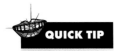
QUICK TIP

With less than ten minutes a day, we can help our children build self-esteem and set the course for a lifetime of cavity-free teeth.

neighbors, teachers, peers and other family members.

In our society, impressions count. Children who have a clean, white smile are more likely to feel good about themselves and be welcomed by others. They will feel comfortable in social settings and speak with fewer inhibitions than children who have black decay marks, bad breath or teeth growing in the wrong direction.

As parents, we want to help our children to be their best, inside and out. Achieving a beautiful smile is a relatively simple accomplishment. With less than ten minutes a day, we can help our children build self-esteem and learn healthy dental habits.

In the following chapters we will discuss why teeth are attacked by dental decay. I will explain how dental and oral bacteria work, which bacteria are bad, how we can reduce the amount of bad bacteria, and how we can minimize the damage caused by the bacteria.

I will show you how you can maximize the tooth's resistance to make your children's teeth stronger, using easy techniques at home. And I will offer suggestions for treatments which your dentist can provide that are proven, sure-fire ways of stopping decay.

There is no reason why your child can't have great looking teeth that function well, enhance good speech development and aid in the process of optimum nutrition. Let's go on to discuss what we can do to prevent decay and set the groundwork for maintaining a lifetime of healthy smiles.

THE BENEFITS OF CAVITY PREVENTION

CHAPTER TWO

The Battle Between Teeth And Bacteria

Most children eat three meals plus three snacks daily. That means that the average child is exposed to acid on their tooth enamel for at least two hours every day.

Before I explain the details of my cavity prevention program, I think it's useful to explain just what cavities are and what causes them. To illustrate, I'll use the A, B, C model of tooth decay, which emphasizes the crucial point that cavities result from a combination of three basic elements:

A= TOOTH
B= BACTERIA
C= CARBOHYDRATES

Stated simply, a cavity is formed when certain bacteria are present on the tooth and there are carbohydrates available for the bacteria to consume. As the bacteria consume the carbohydrates, an acid is produced that dissolves the

THE BATTLE BETWEEN TEETH AND BACTERIA

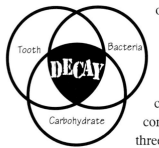

outside coating of the tooth, and the result is a cavity. If you take away any one of these three elements - tooth, bacteria or carbohydrate - you take away the possibility for a cavity. Since we really cannot take away any of these three components, we must work to control all three to prevent decay for our children.

A: TEETH

In discussing how to protect teeth and keep them strong, it is useful to understand the composition of teeth.

Teeth are made up of three parts: enamel, dentin and pulp. The enamel is the outer protective layer, a white coating that is very strong and dense. Dentin is the middle layer that is not as hard, and more yellow. The pulp is the center, the nerve, and the blood supply of the tooth.

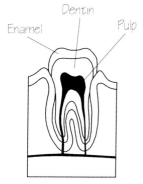

Because enamel is the outer layer, it is the part of the tooth we can most easily reach and protect. To help the enamel do its job, we need to provide daily protection and care.

BRICKS AND MORTAR

If we could examine enamel under a microscope, it would look like a brick wall with mortar holding the bricks in place. Now, imagine a wall where the mortar starts to dissolve and some of the bricks fall out. This is how a tooth decays. If the pH, which is a measure of acidity and

CHAPTER TWO

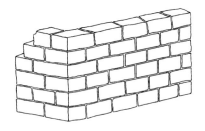

Enamel is a lot like a brick wall.

alkalinity, reaches an excessively acidic level for a lengthy period of time, some of the mortar begins to dissolve. When too much mortar is lost, bricks start to fall out.

We've all seen solid walls break down, usually due to damaging elements such as weather. Teeth break down in much the same way. The acidic pH that causes tooth decay results from bacterial action in our mouths. When certain bacteria are fed with foods such as sugar or starch, acid that dissolves tooth enamel is quickly produced. This dissolving acid may create a hole. Once started, bacteria will move into the hole, hiding from brushing and flossing. The bacteria produce more acid and dissolve more tooth substance. This is the way decay works on a tooth.

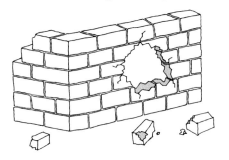

A decayed tooth is like a brick wall with weak mortar and missing bricks.

The goal for us as parents then, is to strengthen our children's enamel as much as possible. If we can keep all the bricks, so to speak, in place and not allow the mortar to dissolve, we will keep our children's teeth solid and decay-free.

B: BACTERIA

Bacteria are one-celled organisms that are involved in fermentation, putrefaction, infectious diseases or nitrogen fixation, according to the Random House Dictionary.

Many different types of bacteria live in our mouth,

some good, some not-so-good. One type of not-so-good bacteria is Strep mutans.

These bacteria are located primarily on the outer layer of the teeth. When in the presence of a fermentable carbohydrate such as sucrose (sugar), Strep mutans can cause an acidification of dental plaque. If the acidic levels in the saliva reach a pH level of 5.2 or lower, (7.0 is neutral), tooth enamel can demineralize. The lower the pH, the higher the acidic level - meaning that the potential for tooth enamel to demineralize, becomes greater.

Stated in another way, parts of your child's tooth will be lost like bricks and mortar being worn away. If a tooth is assaulted by this bacterial acid for an extended period of time, a hole will develop in the tooth's enamel wall. The bacteria will now start to grow in this hole and keep dissolving into the next layer of the tooth, thus forming a cavity.

Bacteria, when given a carbohydrate such as candy, will use the sugar to feed upon. With each exposure to these carbohydrates, bacteria produce acid for about 20 minutes. Most children eat three meals plus three snacks daily. That means that the average child is exposed to acid on their tooth enamel for at least two hours every day.

Most of the time, teeth can handle the assault of this acid, using natural defenses found in the saliva. However, if there is an overwhelming presence of bacteria, or plaque, problems may arise due to excessively high levels of this destructive acid.

LOWERING BACTERIA LEVELS

To help protect your child's teeth, you need to alter the bacterial component in some way. Research is in progress to produce a vaccine for Strep mutans, but a satisfactory result has not yet been reached.

In the meantime, there are a number of useful

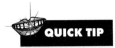

QUICK TIP

One of the most important goals of brushing and flossing is not just to get the food your child has eaten off the teeth, but to actually decrease amounts of damaging bacteria from the surface of the teeth.

techniques you can use to decrease the amount of cavity-forming bacteria in your child's mouth.

Try to keep your child's teeth as bacteria-free as possible, with methods such as brushing, flossing or wiping. These are discussed in detail in Chapter Four. One of the most important goals of brushing and flossing is not just to get the food off the teeth, but to actually decrease the amount of damaging bacteria on the surface of the teeth.

Brushing three times a day is an important habit that keeps the amount and concentrations of bacteria low, so the acid levels are also low. The importance of good oral hygiene is impossible to overstate, since it is a major component in keeping bacteria at bay.

C: CARBOHYDRATES

Carbohydrates are a necessary food group for our children's healthy growth and development. However, there are good and bad carbohydrates and we need to know what they are and how they work.

So-called "simple" carbohydrates such as candy, cookies and sweet cereals have a relatively simple biochemical structure. This means that they are quickly and easily broken down (digested) into their component parts (sugars). The process of digestion begins in the mouth as soon as the carbohydrate foods are mixed with saliva - making the sugars immediately available to oral bacteria. As we know, this will result in acid production that is harmful to the teeth.

Complex carbohydrates, such as grains

THE BATTLE BETWEEN TEETH AND BACTERIA

and vegetables, have a more complicated biochemical structure. These foods take longer to break down, as they require acids found in the stomach. Because complex carbohydrates are not significantly digested by the relatively weak action of saliva, the oral bacteria is deprived of the component sugar they need for fuel. Therefore there is less production of the enamel dissolving acid in the mouth.

Chapter Five provides a more detailed explanation of carbohydrates and the role they can play in cavity prevention or production.

CHAPTER THREE

The Dangers Of Tooth Decay

In many instances, infant cavities

can lead to problems down the road that

are much more easily avoided than fixed.

"BUT DOCTOR, THEY'RE JUST BABY
TEETH. WHY SHOULD I WORRY?"

Past generations may have shrugged
off concerns about cavities in baby teeth.
Well-meaning friends and relatives may
have said, "Don't worry, baby teeth fall out
and your little boy or girl will get new
teeth soon." Guess what? They were
wrong.

Cavity prevention should begin with
infants. Picture the tiny teeth of a baby.
Those little teeth have roots in the jaw
and inside these roots are nerves and
blood vessels, which in turn connect
these baby teeth to the brain, the heart
and to the rest of the body. It stands to
reason that we want to avoid a potential
connection between a bacterial infection
(cavity) and these vital organs.

THE DANGERS OF TOOTH DECAY

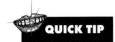

QUICK TIP

If you feel the need to put a bottle in bed with your child, please use only plain water. If you nurse or feed your baby to sleep, please clean his or her teeth and gums with a damp cloth or small, soft-bristle toothbrush. Usually, this will not wake your child and the healthy benefits are tremendous.

It's very important to realize that baby bottle decay is a serious condition, but it can be easily avoided by the use of this very simple tip.

In many instances, infant cavities can lead to problems down the road that are much more easily avoided than fixed. If decay reaches the pulp area, then an infection inside the tooth will cause pain to your child. This usually results in an unhappy child (and justifiably so!) who is kept awake at night and is fussy during the day because of discomfort and pain. If an abscess occurs in a baby tooth, the permanent tooth may be damaged in the course of the infection, causing it to be misshapen, or marked by unsightly white, yellow or brown spotting. An abscessed baby tooth may also cause a permanent tooth to change its normal path of eruption.

BABY BOTTLE DECAY

You may have heard of a special type of decay called nursing bottle decay or baby bottle decay. I believe it deserves special mention as it is so destructive.

In my career, I have performed surgery on more than a thousand infants, with tooth decay because of bedtime bottles or breast feeding on demand, without having their teeth cleaned afterwards. I have also treated many two- and three-year-old patients who have had all of their 20 teeth destroyed by decay. These infants and toddlers have to undergo general anesthesia for extractions and repairs that could easily have been avoided.

Infant tooth decay typically arises when a child goes to sleep with a bottle in the crib or bed. It can also occur when baby gums and

CHAPTER THREE

teeth are not cleaned after bottle or breast feeding. The sugars found in milk or juice work on the baby's teeth while they are sleeping. Saliva, a natural buffer against acid, is less present in the baby's mouth during sleep, and the result is that acids continue to be produced in greater amounts and can exert their destructive effects for a longer period of time.

This acid is dangerous because it dissolves enamel. Initial findings of baby bottle decay may include whitish lines forming on the teeth, usually along the gum line. Later symptoms include cavities and infection.

You can accomplish so much towards achieving good dental health for your infant with this simple bit of advice. Baby bottle decay is so unnecessary and you can easily prevent it from happening to your child.

Tooth And Consequences

If you have had cavities, you understand the pain associated with them. You also know how it feels to have one repaired. For those few and lucky parents who do not know, believe me, you do not want your child to get dental decay if possible.

Even in cases where pain is not severe, decay can lead to chronic discomfort. Sometimes, a two- or three-year-old child will not have the verbal skills to tell us they are feeling pain. They may even believe the pain to be a normal sensation and simply live with it since they don't know any better. Such an oversight could lead to years of dental problems.

Abscessed Teeth

If decay progresses into the inner pulp area and the infection is left untreated, the inside of the tooth becomes rotten and produces pus. This condition is called an abscess. It is potentially damaging and in certain

THE DANGERS OF TOOTH DECAY

circumstances, even life-threatening.

An abscess results when pus from the tooth causes bone in the jaw to dissolve as it looks for an avenue of escape. Symptoms of this condition often include swelling of the cheek, chin, eye, lip or gum. Antibiotics are generally prescribed to control the swelling, but medication cannot cure the infection. The infection can only be cured by cleaning out the inside of the tooth, usually with a root canal, or by extracting the tooth.

During the course of this infection, the permanent tooth, which sits at the root tip of the baby tooth, may become damaged or develop unsightly white, yellow or brown spotting as well as pitting or odd shaping. Infection can also cause a permanent tooth to grow in a different direction than it would have normally.

If the bacterial infection in the tooth becomes severe enough, the tooth will become a pus-producing factory. This pus has to go somewhere, and the only path out is through the tip of the root to the bone. While this process may at first be painless, it is a dangerous condition. Once the inside of the tooth is rotten and destroyed, nerve damage may no longer be felt since the nerves have also been destroyed.

An abscessed tooth usually can't be detected just by looking into the mouth. Because of the depth of the infection, x-rays are often required to make a diagnosis. Your child may not even feel any pain while the infection spreads through the bone. But if your child appears to have any of the symptoms described above, or is complaining of pain while chewing, call your dentist immediately.

EARLY EXTRACTIONS

When teeth need to be removed, a whole new set of complications arises. In addition to the trauma of

CHAPTER THREE

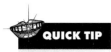
QUICK TIP

I've been performing dental surgery on small children for many years. And I am always struck by a recurring observation from parents. During our follow-up visits, parents quite frequently comment on the remarkable improvement in their child's appetite and eating habits. It never fails to move me how quickly good eating habits develop in young children once an infected tooth is restored or extracted.

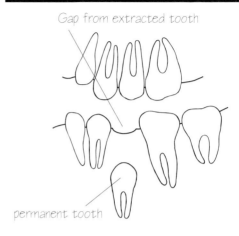

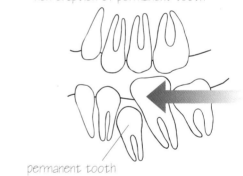

extracting a tooth from an infant, toddler or child, we now have to worry about space being maintained in the jaw to accommodate permanent teeth. If a tooth is lost before its natural time, remaining teeth may drift into the gap, and interfere with natural jaw development and eruption of permanent teeth.

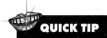

QUICK TIP

See your dentist if your child has any of the following warning signs of infection: Fever, combined with puffiness around the mouth, bleeding or swollen gums, avoiding crunchy or sweet foods, or avoiding or complaining about hot and cold foods or drinks, or whitish lines forming on infant teeth.

Early extractions may even result in an impaction or non-eruption of permanent teeth in the jaw. Once this occurs, braces or surgery may be the only recourse, in an effort to reclaim this space and get the permanent teeth to erupt into the mouth.

OTHER PROBLEMS CAUSED BY INFECTION

Cavities and abscesses may also result in poor nutritional intake. Certain foods may be painful for your child to chew, and so he may stop eating them. Obviously, if your child stops eating nutritious foods, it could affect his normal growth and development.

Even disposition can be affected. The child who lives with constant discomfort will certainly feel unhappy and frustrated by chronic pain.

CHAPTER FOUR

Fighting Back – The War Against Bacteria

We want to stop decay before it begins.

One method is to alter the amounts and activity of

bacteria in our child's mouth.

THE FIRST STEP

The first step is to physically remove the bacteria, or plaque, as it is called once it builds up and creates a sticky home for itself on the tooth. The most effective and easiest way to do this is by regularly brushing and flossing your child's teeth, paying special attention to the gumline of each tooth and chewing surfaces.

A parent should be actively involved in brushing their child's teeth until the ages of eight to ten. Your child may exhibit a gift for independence and self-reliance, but still, they will not be as motivated as you.

Even if they brush for a full three minutes, they really don't have the motor skills required. Just as you would not expect a young child to drive a car or

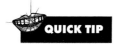

QUICK TIP

The most effective and easily accomplished technique available for removing bacteria is brushing and flossing your child's teeth, especially along the gumline of each tooth and the chewing surfaces.

A parent should be actively involved in brushing their child's teeth until the ages of eight to ten.

cook an omelet, you should not expect them to have the dexterity needed to do a really thorough job of brushing their teeth.

How do you ensure that brushing is a regular part of your child's daily routine? This is where your parenting skills are developed and tested. Some children take to brushing instantly, while others fight it three times a day. But with a little creative thinking, you can make brushing a fun activity.

One of the easiest ways is to be a good role model. If your children see you brushing your teeth for a full three minutes, they will be inclined to follow your example. Ask your dentist and other parents for suggestions. Be prepared to come up with new ideas as your child grows. (See suggestions at the end of this chapter)

What Age Should You Start Brushing And Cleaning?

Even if your infant has only one tooth, it is time to start fighting off bacteria. Get in the habit of wiping baby teeth and gums with a damp, clean cloth at least three times a day, or after every feeding.

One of the most important times to clean teeth is before sleep, when saliva production decreases. Saliva is a natural buffer that counters the acids produced by bacteria. If your child goes to sleep without having her teeth cleaned, the acids will be able to do more damage to the enamel over a greater period of time.

CHAPTER FOUR

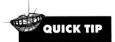
QUICK TIP

Remember, teeth have three surfaces that need brushing:
1. Inside Surface
2. Chewing or Top Surface
3. Outside or Lip Cheek Surface

When brushing the outside surface of teeth, have your child close his mouth almost all the way. This will make it easier for you to stretch the lip and cheek away and thoroughly clean the outside surfaces of the teeth.

Now, have your child open wide and brush the chewing surfaces and visually inspect inside the mouth for any food remnants. If you see any white build-up on the tongue, you should try to brush this as well, but don't go too far back or you may cause your child to gag.

Finally, do the inside surfaces of the teeth last as this is usually the least favorite part.

HOW TO BRUSH

Now, on to the brushing itself. In brushing your child's teeth, you need to be aware of the area where the gum lies over the tooth. This gum-tooth junction is one to three millimeters deep. It is important to get the toothbrush bristles into this small area in order to clean out bacteria that live there.

JAB, JIGGLE AND ROLL

In dental school we're taught the jab, jiggle and roll theme. Gently jab the bristles down towards the gum line of the teeth, then jiggle them. Roll the toothbrush in the same direction as the teeth are growing. After doing this to all of the teeth, inside and outside, you can scrub them horizontally, side to side, or in circles.

This should be done a minimum of two times a day, especially after breakfast and before bed. Three times a day is even better.

Try to brush for a full three minutes. I'm waiting for someone to come up with a singing toothbrush that plays a song for three minutes, to keep our children brushing. There's a hint for an inventor.

FLOSSING & WATER IRRIGATION DEVICES

Flossing should start when teeth begin to touch each other and the areas between cannot be reached with a toothbrush. Once begun, flossing should be continued daily. If your child rejects floss, you can try using a water irrigation device that flushes debris off teeth. Although water irrigation devices are not a total replacement for brushing and flossing, they can be an important aid, especially for children who wear braces. Sometimes your dentist may recommend that you use a special bacterial reducing solution with the water irrigation device. As with brushing, flossing will be most effective if done before going to sleep, when the saliva flow decreases.

How To Floss

• Tear off a long piece of floss. Pinch one end between your left thumb and another finger. Wrap floss around that finger three turns. Now do the same with your right hand and wrap floss until you have a 4" length between your thumb tips.

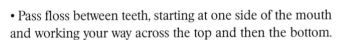

• Pass floss between teeth, starting at one side of the mouth and working your way across the top and then the bottom.

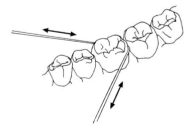

Slide the floss between two teeth with movement inside and out, until you feel it pass between the contact area of the two teeth. Wrap floss in a c-shape around the tooth and remember to clean two teeth with each pass of floss.

• Always move floss gently up and down between teeth and the delicate gum space.

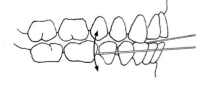

CHAPTER FOUR

• Pull floss out and go on to the next teeth. Adjust floss between hands if it becomes dirty or frayed.

• Remember that flossing only needs to be done when teeth are touching.

• If you find that your floss is shredding, try one of the teflon flosses now available.

• You may also choose to try a floss holder. This is a Y-shaped device that keeps the floss tight, instead of using fingers. Many find the floss holder easier to maneuver.

• There are different types of floss such as ribbon, tape, flavored and teflon. I have found that my children enjoy the flavored tape floss over all others.

WHICH TOOTHPASTE TO USE?

There is an excellent selection of fluoridated toothpaste available on the market. I strongly recommend using a brand that is stamped with the seal of approval from the American Dental Association. This identifies that the toothpaste has been clinically studied and that it not only contains fluoride, but the fluoride is properly released onto the tooth. When choosing flavors or colors, find a toothpaste your child most enjoys using. My children have each always preferred using different toothpastes and you can bet I buy different types to keep them happy and brushing.

WHICH TOOTHBRUSH TO CHOOSE?

With the large selection of toothbrushes available, you and your child should have no trouble finding one you both like. Look for two basic features that will help you achieve optimum results.

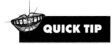

QUICK TIP

When brushing your child's teeth, please pay special attention to the amount of toothpaste you use.

Only use a pea size or smaller amount of toothpaste and have your child spit out any extra as soon as he is able. You do not want your child to ingest too much fluoride on a daily basis, as he may develop a condition called fluorosis. Fluorosis can cause permanent blemishes on the teeth that will not fade over time. (see page 47)

1. The size of the toothbrush should be appropriate for your child's mouth. If the toothbrush head is too large, there will not be room for it to move and scrubbing activity will be less effective. If the toothbrush head is too small, certain areas of the teeth will be missed. I recommend a child-size brush, as do most of the dentists and dental hygienists I know.

2. Look also for a toothbrush with a rounded head that has soft, polished bristles. Cleansing action is primarily achieved through the mechanical action of the brush, water and detergents in the toothpaste. Hard bristles do not clean any better and may in fact, damage gum tissue. Electric toothbrushes are very good and will do a thorough job. But they will also increase your costs, and some can be used only with their own brand of toothpaste and/or replaceable heads.

How Often Should A Toothbrush Be Replaced?

The general rule of thumb is that if bristles are splaying, spreading out or feeling soft, it's time for a new brush. I recommend replacing toothbrushes every three to six months or sooner if your child has had an oral infection or strep throat.

Letting a child choose her own toothbrush is a great way to keep your child involved in dental care. Have fun choosing and using new child-oriented brushes. Some feature television or movie characters, others glow-in-the-dark and still others have handles

CHAPTER FOUR

that change color or make noises.

As a pediatric dentist and father of young children, I've learned that if we can make the task fun, we win most of the battles before they begin.

ANTI-BACTERIAL RINSES

Another way we can lower the amount of bacteria in our child's mouth is with an anti-bacterial rinse. These are readily available by prescription and as over-the-counter products in the pharmacy or supermarket.

Although rinses can be very effective for reducing the amounts of damaging bacteria, they should only be used after consulting with your child's dentist. Some of these rinses can alter taste or stain your child's teeth. Some also contain ingredients such as ethanol, that your child should not ingest.

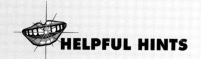

HELPFUL HINTS

How To Encourage Your Child To Brush

- Let children choose attractive toothbrushes
- Choose a flavored toothpaste that your child enjoys
- Play a tape or sing a three-minute brushing song
- Use a three-minute wind up toy while brushing
- Brush in a different location, such as the bathtub or kitchen
- Keep a toothbrush in more than one bathroom for in-between brushings
- Use a three-minute hourglass-style egg timer

CHAPTER FIVE

Food – The Good, The Bad & The Ugly

Some foods actually have a cleansing effect

on teeth and are believed to help inhibit decay

through an anti-bacterial effect.

FEEDING HEALTHY TEETH

As your children grow older and begin to eat regular meals and snacks, it is important to be aware of how certain foods will affect their teeth. As a general rule, sticky, processed, highly refined and retentive foods, are not good. By retentive, I mean those that stick to teeth or get wedged in between teeth for long periods of time. Foods that are safer for teeth include those that are fibrous and don't stay in the mouth long.

Simple sugars, such as sucrose, refined sugars and corn syrup are dangerous because they are a major source of food for bacteria. Sticky foods such as gummy-type candies or processed fruit snacks are even more dangerous because they get stuck in areas

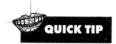

QUICK TIP

When I meet parents of new patients, one of the first pieces of advice I give is to avoid all gummy-type candies as well as sticky fruit snacks.

These gummy types of snacks have extremely destructive properties and have become a prime cause of cavities for young children.

Although often marketed as healthful because of their high fruit content, these products are simple, refined carbohydrates that are extremely difficult to remove from teeth.

In my practice, I see thousands of children each year, who despite good brushing habits, develop cavities as a result of snacking on gummy and fruit snack treats.

where they cannot easily be removed with a toothbrush.

In addition to avoiding sticky, gummy-type candies, also try to avoid dried fruits, potato chips, sweetened cereals, cookies and other retentive foods. Crumbly foods that get stuck in grooves or between teeth are also more likely to cause cavities.

GOOD FOOD CHOICES

On the good foods list are fibrous or quick-dissolving foods such as raw fruits, raw vegetables, pretzels, popcorn and other non-retentive or quickly clearing foods. Some foods actually have a cleansing effect on teeth, and are believed to help inhibit decay through an anti-bacterial effect. These foods include milk, cheese and oats. Please note that though certain foods have a positive effect on teeth, it is still advisable to maintain good brushing habits after meals.

CARBOHYDRATES AND TEETH

Carbohydrates are an important food group that our children need to grow and be healthy. Again, there are good and bad carbohydrates. Among those that are damaging to our children's teeth are sugar and sucrose. These simple sugars are readily utilized by mouth bacteria and result in increased acid production.

Other sugars actually seem to fight decay. Sorbitol, a sweetener found in certain sugarless gums, has been shown to be effective in warding off decay, although in

CHAPTER FIVE

large doses may cause diarrhea.

GOOD CARBOHYDRATES

On the good list of food choices are complex carbohydrates. These foods offer nutritional benefits and are not as great a threat to teeth. Because they take more time to break down, harmful acids are not produced in the mouth since they are primarily digested and broken down in the stomach. Vegetables and grains are good foods to consider when trying to avoid decay.

FOOD - THE GOOD, THE BAD & THE UGLY

Good Snacks That Won't Hurt Your Teeth
Salted Nuts, Popcorn, Apples, Oranges, Bananas, Celery, Baby Carrots, Red & Green Pepper Slices, Radishes, Plums, Cucumber Slices, Cantaloupe, Pickles, Melon, Hard Cheese, Meat Slices, Hard-Boiled Eggs, Diabetic Soft Drinks and Diabetic Foods

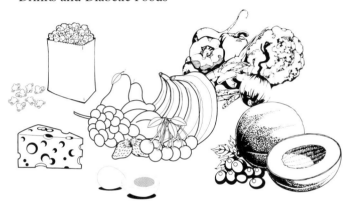

Bad Snacks That Could Hurt Your Teeth
Gummy Candies, Hard Candies, Dried Fruits, Soda Pop, Ice Cream, Cookies, Cake, Pie, Popsicles, Sweet Rolls, Caramel Popcorn, Crackers (graham or soda), Gelatin Desserts, Peanut Butter Sandwiches, Potato Chips anything sticky, sweet or starchy (e.g. white bread)

CHAPTER FIVE

Sugar Content In Breakfast Cereals

This list gives the sugar content (in grams), of a variety of popular breakfast cereals.

Cereal Product Name	Grams of Sugar in a one-ounce serving
Nutri-grain Corn Cereal	0
Shredded Wheat	0
Puffed Rice	0
Spoon Size Shredded Wheat	0
Cheerios	1
Wheat Chex	2
Rice Chex	2
Nutri-grain Barley Cereal	2
Crispix	3
Concentrate Cereal	3
Rice Krispies	3
Grape Nuts	3
Corn Flakes	3
Product 19	3
Special K	3
Corn Total	3
Smart Start for Women	4
All-Bran Cereal	5
Buc Wheats	5
Toasted Wheat & Raisins	5
Bran Chex	5
Pep Cereal	5
Fortified Oat Flakes	6
Corn Bran	6
100% Natural Cereal	6
Life Cereal	6
40% Bran Flakes	6
Kaboom	6
King Vitamin	6
Cinnamon Life	6
100% Bran	6
Fruit & Fiber w/Apples & Cinnamon	7
Toasted Mini Wheats	7
Bran Buds	7
Country Morning	7
Nature Valley Granola	8
Raisin, Rice & Rye	8
Cinnamon Frosted Mini Wheats	8
Most Cereal	8
CW Post with Raisins	8
Cracklin Bran	8
Honey Nut Crunch Raisin Bran	8
Graham Crackos	9

40

FOOD - THE GOOD, THE BAD & THE UGLY

Sugar Content In Breakfast Cereals (cont'd)

Cereal Product Name	Grams of Sugar in a one-ounce serving
100% Natural Cereal w/Raisins & Dates	9
Post Raisin Bran	9
Country Morning w/Raisins & Dates	9
Cinnamon Toast Crunch	9
Golden Grahams	10
Crispy Wheat & Raisins	10
Honey Nut Cheerios	10
ET	10
Gremlins	10
Wheat Raisin Chex	10
Marshmallow Krispies	10
Raisin Bran	11
Lucky Charms	11
Body Buddies	11
Alpha Bits	11
Cocoa Puffs	11
Honey Comb	11
C-3PO's	11
Cap'n Crunch	12
Cocoa Krispies	12
Trix	12
Pacman	12
Donkey Kong	12
Crispy Oatmeal & Raisin Chex	12
Apple Raisin Crisp	12
Frosted Flakes of Corn	13
Sugar Corn Pops	13
Fruit Loops	13
Cocoa Krispies	13
Frankenberry	13
Frosted Rice	13
Count Chocula	13
Cookie Crisp	13
Donkey Kong Junior	13
Cap'n Crunch's Choco Crunch	13
Raisin Life	13
Cap'n Crunch Crunch Berries	13
Smurf Berry Crunch	13
Fruity Pebbles	13
Cocoa Pebbles	13
Rainbow Brite	14
Apple Jacks	15
Sugar Smacks	15
Honey Smacks	16

Source: Patricia Thonney, Extension Associate Cornell University, Ithaca, NY

CHAPTER FIVE

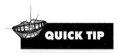
QUICK TIP

HALLOWEEN TRICK: Here's an idea I used this year with my children. After a fun night of dressing in costumes and trick-or-treating, I made them a proposition: I would pay for all their candy and take them to a toy store the following day so that they could choose whatever their candy earnings would buy. One child was sold on the idea right away; the other had to mull it over for a couple of minutes, but soon decided to take the money and go for the toy.

Frequency Of Meals And Snacks

The other important element of diet is frequency of eating. If your children are snacking all day on raisins, cereal or other carbohydrates, the acid level in their mouths will be high, and they will be more susceptible to dental decay for a longer period of time.

Try to establish regular eating times in the day. When meals and snacks are spaced out, tooth enamel destruction does not become a constant process, and the body has resources to protect itself.

Of course, you can't always deny children snacks and treats. But do try to use extra caution when brushing and flossing after sticky, retentive foods are eaten. Also, try not to give sweet snacks randomly throughout the day. Instead offer sweets after meal times when other refined carbohydrates are already being consumed, and teeth are likely to be brushed afterwards. Then you can offer raw or unprocessed healthy snacks between meals to minimize acid production.

Extra Snacks = Extra Acid

Remember, if your child eats three meals a day plus three snacks a day, this will usually result in about two hours of acid production from their oral bacteria, as there is approximately 20 minutes of acid produced with each carbohydrate exposure.

FOOD - THE GOOD, THE BAD & THE UGLY

If you add three or four more "snack or treat times," you will be adding another hour or more of acid exposure. And – if the snack is a highly refined or retentive type of carbohydrate, this danger zone will be even greater!

CHAPTER SIX

Giving Nature A Hand - Techniques To Protect And Strengthen Teeth

Our goal as parents is to make the enamel on our children's teeth as strong as possible, so it can resist acids that lead to cavity production.

As we have seen, it is the enamel - the outer layer - of the tooth that guards against the invasion of harmful bacteria. Our goal as parents is to make the enamel on our children's teeth as strong as possible, so it can resist acids that lead to cavity production. The cavity prevention part of this program is an area where your child's dentist can be a tremendous ally.

THE FLUORIDE CONNECTION

Teeth begin growing and continue forming in the jawbone as your child develops, from in utero right through to their teens. Once a tooth appears in the mouth, it is already fully calcified, and the enamel stops growing.

44

Fluoride benefits the tooth in two ways.

1. When fluoride is ingested through drinking water, other beverages or a fluoride supplement, teeth developing in the jaw become stronger and more resistant to decay.

2. Once teeth erupt and fluoride is applied topically with toothpaste, rinses or fluoride treatments, the enamel becomes more resistant to bacteria, acid and decay.

FLUORIDE TREATMENTS

The best way to keep enamel from dissolving is to make it more resistant to acid. Tooth enamel starts off with a very high concentration of fluoride in its outer layers. This fluoride can dissolve away over time if it is constantly exposed to acidic pH. We can help keep teeth strong by keeping the enamel's fluoride level up to its maximum strength.

Here's an example: In a swimming pool, you need to keep up the chlorine level so that bacteria and algae do not contaminate the water. First the pool is "shocked" with a massive dose of chlorine. Over the season, more is added in smaller, regular doses to maintain an optimum level. Along with these regular additions, it is still necessary to "shock" the pool occasionally with larger amounts of chlorine, to keep bacteria away.

Teeth are similar. That is why when your child goes to the dentist, it is highly advisable that he receives a topical fluoride treatment. Applied directly to your child's teeth, the fluoride is of a very high concentration. It replenishes the enamel supply, bringing it back to its optimum strength.

Your child should receive a topical fluoride treatment from his dentist at least two times a year. Fluoride treatments are applied quickly and easily and come in a variety of child-friendly flavors. These treatments, along with other sources of fluoride, will greatly improve your

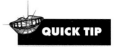

QUICK TIP

Your child should receive topical fluoride treatments from his or her dentist at least two times a year. This, along with other sources of fluoride, will greatly improve your effort in stopping cavities from developing on the smooth surfaces of teeth.

efforts in stopping cavities from forming on the smooth surfaces of your child's teeth.

Over time the fluoride will leach out, so it is important to add more topically on a daily basis. This is easily achieved by using a fluoridated toothpaste. Your dentist may even suggest the use of a fluoride rinse, fluoride gel or a fluoride varnish that is painted onto teeth to give a long, slow release of fluoride to the enamel.

Please Note: the amount of fluoride that is needed varies according to the size and age of the child. Before starting a child on a rinse or a gel, a dentist should always be consulted.

Fluoride In Drinking Water

When fluoride is ingested or swallowed before teeth grow in, the teeth will be stronger and more resistant to decay.

There are many ways to ingest fluoride. One of the most effective is to drink fluoridated water. Many communities have already added fluoride to their drinking water, an effort that has been incredibly successful in cavity reduction.

If you live in an area where there is no fluoridation of the drinking water, you should consult with the child's physician or dentist to see if they recommend a dietary fluoride supplement. Such supplements are available by prescription and can help developing teeth grow in with a much greater resistance to decay.

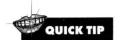

QUICK TIP

Swallowing too much fluoridated toothpaste on a regular basis is a cause of fluorosis. Remember that only a pea-size amount of toothpaste (or less) should be used for all children. Don't allow children to eat toothpaste or apply toothpaste to their own toothbrush until they are old enough to understand how much to use. Always encourage your child to rinse and spit out excess toothpaste.

FLUOROSIS

Although fluoride offers many benefits, too much can have damaging effects. A certain amount will help form stronger enamel, but if your child ingests excessive quantities, a condition called fluorosis may develop.

Fluorosis occurs while teeth are still forming in the jaw and primarily affects children from infancy to twelve years of age. Excessive ingestion of fluoride can cause permanent tooth blemishes which are usually brown, yellow or chalky white, giving the tooth a mottled or dirty look that will not fade away.

Swallowing too much toothpaste on a regular basis is an avoidable cause of fluorosis. Remember that only a pea-size amount of toothpaste should be used for all children less than six years of age. Most children are prone to eating more toothpaste than they should. For this reason it is very important that you never allow your child to eat toothpaste. Always encourage your child to rinse and spit out excess toothpaste.

It's important to talk to your dentist about whether the right amount of fluoride is being ingested, while your child is still an infant. Remember – in addition to drinking water, most reconstituted beverages are made with fluoridated water. This includes commercially available formula, fruit juices, sodas, and even quite a few bottled waters.

CHAPTER SIX

DENTAL SEALANTS

Topical fluoride treatments are great for protecting the smooth parts of teeth. The chewing surfaces of the back teeth present a different challenge. Eighty percent of all cavities occur in children's back teeth where grooves and pits on the chewing surfaces trap food and harbor bacteria. These grooves are so narrow that our toothbrushes often cannot reach down to the bottom. Bacteria that cause decay hide in these grooves, as do sugars and carbohydrates.

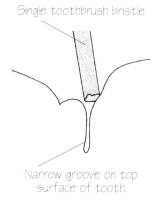

Fortunately, these areas can easily be protected by your dentist. If your child's teeth have deep narrow grooves, a sealant may be recommended. Dental sealants form a barrier between the tooth enamel and bacteria. If the bacteria and their acids cannot touch the tooth, a cavity will not form. Sealants are a powerful tool in cavity prevention, especially for parts of the teeth which have pits or grooves, and cannot easily be cleaned with a toothbrush, floss or rinse.

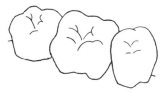
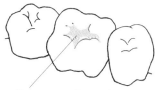

Another benefit of sealants is that they are applied quickly and painlessly. No drilling or Novocaine™ is required. Some sealants contain fluoride which is slowly released over time. Sealants can be clear or colored.

To apply a sealant, the tooth is cleansed and prepared for the liquid resin which is flowed into the grooves and quickly bonded to the tooth.

Once grooves and pits are converted to a smooth surface, bacteria and carbohydrates cannot get into the grooves and affect the enamel. Teeth with sealants can also be cleaned more effectively with a toothbrush.

Sealants have been shown to stop more than 80% of dental decay within two years of placement. They offer a great, painless option when looking for ways to reduce cavities for your child.

How Sealants Prevent Cavities

- Eighty percent of all cavities occur in children's back teeth where grooves and pits on the chewing surfaces trap food and harbor bacteria.

- Dental sealants form a barrier between the enamel and bacteria. If the bacteria and their acids cannot touch the tooth, a cavity will not form.

- Sealants have been shown to stop more than 80% of dental decay within two years of the placement. They offer a great, painless option when looking for ways to reduce cavities for your child.

Partnership With Your Dentist

By working effectively with your child's dentist and dental hygienist, you can eliminate cavities for your child. Every dentist I know would love to see your child stay

CHAPTER SIX

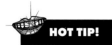
HOT TIP!

CHECK-OUT our web site at: www.lookmom.com – for updates in new advances in preventing decay. We change our information as new research is reported. We also add helpful hints. If you have some helpful ideas you would like to share, please e-mail us at: pdcpress@lookmom.com

cavity-free forever and will be happy to work with you to achieve this goal.

New advances in dentistry are constantly being developed. Your dentist is your link to learning more about emerging methods as well as preventative and restorative techniques. Your dental hygienist can also offer many informative suggestions.

FIRST DENTAL VISIT

A first dental visit should take place around one year of age although there are exceptions. As I mentioned earlier, I have seen far too many 12- to 18-month-old children who have had to undergo general anesthesia because of early decay. I recommend bringing your child to the dentist for a "look-see" and consultation upon eruption of the first tooth.

GIVING NATURE A HAND

CHAPTER SEVEN

Conclusion:
Making Our Goal A Reality

Our goal is to keep our children cavity-free with techniques that will save time and money. Your child will benefit from a healthy smile that will make him or her look and feel good.

PUTTING OUR PLAN INTO ACTION

I promised in my opening letter that I would provide a simple and effective program to help you raise cavity-free children.

THE MAIN ELEMENTS OF THIS PROGRAM INCLUDE:

1. Physically remove harmful bacteria and food particles from the teeth and mouth.
2. Eat foods that do not promote tooth decay.
3. Strengthen the tooth's natural physical barriers.
4. Develop an ongoing relationship with your child's dentist.

CONCLUSION

• We must also remember the three factors that are necessary for decay: tooth, bacteria, and carbohydrates.

• We need to make brushing and flossing fun, regular parts of our child's day.

• We need to find creative ways to let our children be part of our plan, encouraging them to choose their own appealing toothbrushes and toothpaste.

• We need to watch what and when our children eat, ensuring that their diet aids in our efforts to keep acid production down. We need to avoid sticky and highly processed foods and offer more raw, natural, fibrous and quick-dissolving foods that keep teeth healthy.

• And we need to help make our children's teeth stronger with daily doses of fluoride that are ingested and applied topically with fluoridated toothpaste or rinses. Visiting your child's dentist for fluoride treatments and sealants will make it even more difficult for bacteria to begin the decay process.

• These techniques will save you time and money and your child will benefit from a healthy smile that will make him or her look and feel good. You'll feel good too.

CHAPTER SEVEN

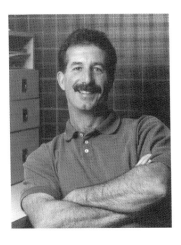

I wish you well in raising a cavity-free child. If you would like to see a video tape showing you specific techniques and further discussion of these and other topics, please contact me by filling out the enclosed order form and sending it to: PDC Press Inc., P.O. Box 548, Buffalo, New York, 14231-0548, or fax the order to (716) 633-2435. You can also call toll-free at 1-888-292-1991 between 9am - 5pm Eastern Standard Time or visit us online on our web site at http://www.lookmom.com for regular updates and ideas.

Sincerely,

Gregory F. George, D.D.S.

CONCLUSION

CHAPTER EIGHT

Check List For Cavity Prevention

INFANTS (BIRTH - 24 MONTHS)

THINGS THAT YOUR DENTIST CAN DO:

✓ Visit dentist when first teeth appear for an initial consultation and "look-see." An early first visit will also help your child become familiar with the dental office and equipment and reduce fears that may develop in toddlers.

✓ Fluoride supplements may be prescribed by a dentist.

CHECK LIST FOR CAVITY PREVENTION

THINGS THAT PARENTS AND CAREGIVERS CAN DO:

☑ Wipe baby gums or teeth with a clean washcloth or gauze pad or toothbrush at least three times a day, after feedings, snacks and always before bedtime.

☑ Avoid putting babies and toddlers to bed with a bottle of milk or juice. If you must use a bedtime bottle, fill it with water only.

☑ Change toothbrush every 3-6 months.

CHAPTER EIGHT

Check List For Cavity Prevention

CHILDREN 2 - 6 YEARS

THINGS THAT YOUR DENTIST CAN DO:

☑ Sealants (a protective coating that covers deep grooves in back teeth) may be recommended.

☑ Fluoride supplements and or treatments may be recommended.

☑ Fluoride Varnish, if required.

☑ Complete professional cleaning.

CHECK LIST FOR CAVITY PREVENTION

THINGS THAT PARENTS AND CAREGIVERS CAN DO:

- ✓ Choose a toothbrush that has a rounded head with soft, polished bristles and is the right size for your child's mouth.
- ✓ Brush teeth 3 times daily, for 3-minutes each time.
- ✓ Begin using pea-sized (or less) amount of fluoridated toothpaste and encourage children to rinse and spit after brushing.
- ✓ Begin flossing any teeth that are touching, every night before bedtime.
- ✓ Change toothbrush every 3-6 months.
- ✓ Visit the dentist every 6 months.
- ✓ Be aware of types of foods and frequency of eating.

CHAPTER EIGHT

Check List For Cavity Prevention

CHILDREN 6 - 12 YEARS

THINGS THAT YOUR DENTIST CAN DO:

✓ Sealants for permanent teeth can be provided.

✓ Fluoride supplements and or treatments may be recommended.

✓ Fluoride Varnish, if required.

✓ Complete professional cleaning.

CHECK LIST FOR CAVITY PREVENTION

THINGS THAT PARENTS AND CAREGIVERS CAN DO:

✔ Begin to transfer responsibility of brushing to child between ages 8-10, depending on child's motor skills and motivation.

✔ Begin to transfer responsibility of flossing to child, no earlier than age 10, as flossing is more difficult than brushing.

✔ Brush teeth 3 times daily if possible.

✔ Change toothbrush every 3-6 months.

✔ Visit the dentist every 6 months.

✔ Be aware of types of foods and frequency of eating.

Look Mom... No Cavities!

TOLL-FREE 1-888-292-1991 (9am - 5pm E.S.T.)

Order a Look Mom...No Cavities! book, video or audio cassette now, and practice this easy-to-follow program in cooperation with your child's dentist.

Mail order form to:
PDC Press, Inc.
P.O. Box 548
Buffalo, NY
14231-0548

Phone: 1-888-292-1991
(TOLL FREE 9am - 5pm E.S.T.)

Fax: (716) 633-2435

e-mail: pdcpress@lookmom.com

Name: _____

Address: _____

_____

City: _____

State: _____ Zip: _____

Phone: _____

METHOD OF PAYMENT

☐ CHECK ☐ MONEY ORDER (Make payable to: PDC Press, Inc.)

CHARGE TO: ☐ VISA ☐ MASTERCARD

CARD#: _____ EXP DATE: _____

SIGNATURE: _____

SAVE UP TO $10.00

ORDER ANY TWO(2) FOR ONLY $29.90

A portion of all proceeds to benefit children's charities and dental schools.

☐ **BOOK** _____ #of copies ($16.95 each)

☐ **VIDEO** _____ #of copies ($19.95 each)

☐ **AUDIO TAPE** _____ #of copies ($19.95 each)

Please call our toll-free number for volume discount information.

MERCHANDISE TOTAL _____

(Add 8% for NY Residents only) **TAX** _____

SHIPPING & HANDLING $6.95

TOTAL _____

Look Mom... No Cavities!

TOLL-FREE 1-888-292-1991 (9am - 5pm E.S.T.)

Order a Look Mom...No Cavities! book, video or audio cassette now, and practice this easy-to-follow program in cooperation with your child's dentist.

Mail order form to:
PDC Press, Inc.
P.O. Box 548
Buffalo, NY
14231-0548

Phone: 1-888-292-1991
(TOLL FREE 9am - 5pm E.S.T.)

Fax: (716) 633-2435

e-mail: pdcpress@lookmom.com

Name: _____

Address: _____

_____

City: _____

State: _____ Zip: _____

Phone: _____

METHOD OF PAYMENT

☐ CHECK ☐ MONEY ORDER (Make payable to: PDC Press, Inc.)

CHARGE TO: ☐ VISA ☐ MASTERCARD

CARD#: _____ EXP DATE: _____

SIGNATURE: _____

SAVE UP TO $10.00

ORDER ANY TWO(2) FOR ONLY $29.90

A portion of all proceeds to benefit children's charities and dental schools.

☐ **BOOK** _____ #of copies ($16.95 each)

☐ **VIDEO** _____ #of copies ($19.95 each)

☐ **AUDIO TAPE** _____ #of copies ($19.95 each)

Please call our toll-free number for volume discount information.

MERCHANDISE TOTAL _____

(Add 8% for NY Residents only) **TAX** _____

SHIPPING & HANDLING $6.95

TOTAL _____

ABOUT THE AUTHOR

GREGORY F. GEORGE, D.D.S. grew up on Long Island, New York. He graduated with a Bachelor of Arts degree from the State University of New York College at Potsdam followed by a Doctor of Dental Surgery degree at the School of Dental Medicine at Buffalo. He also completed a two-year residency in Pediatric Dentistry at the Children's Hospital of Buffalo.

Dr. George has a private practice in pediatric dentistry in Williamsville, N.Y. and has taught at the State University of N.Y. at Buffalo School of Dental Medicine for more than ten years in the Pediatric Dental Department. He has also been awarded the Pediatric Dental Award through the School of Dental Medicine at Buffalo. He is on staff at the Children's Hospital of Buffalo, where he performs dental surgeries. He is a member of the American Society of Dentistry for Children, the American Academy of Pediatric Dentists, the American Dental Association, the New York State Dental Association, the Erie County Dental Association and the Western New York Pediatric Dental Society. He is married to a physician and is the proud parent of cavity-free children.